Diabetic Air Fryer Cookbook

Easy and Flavorful

Recipes

for a Healthy Lifestyle

Lilith Ballard

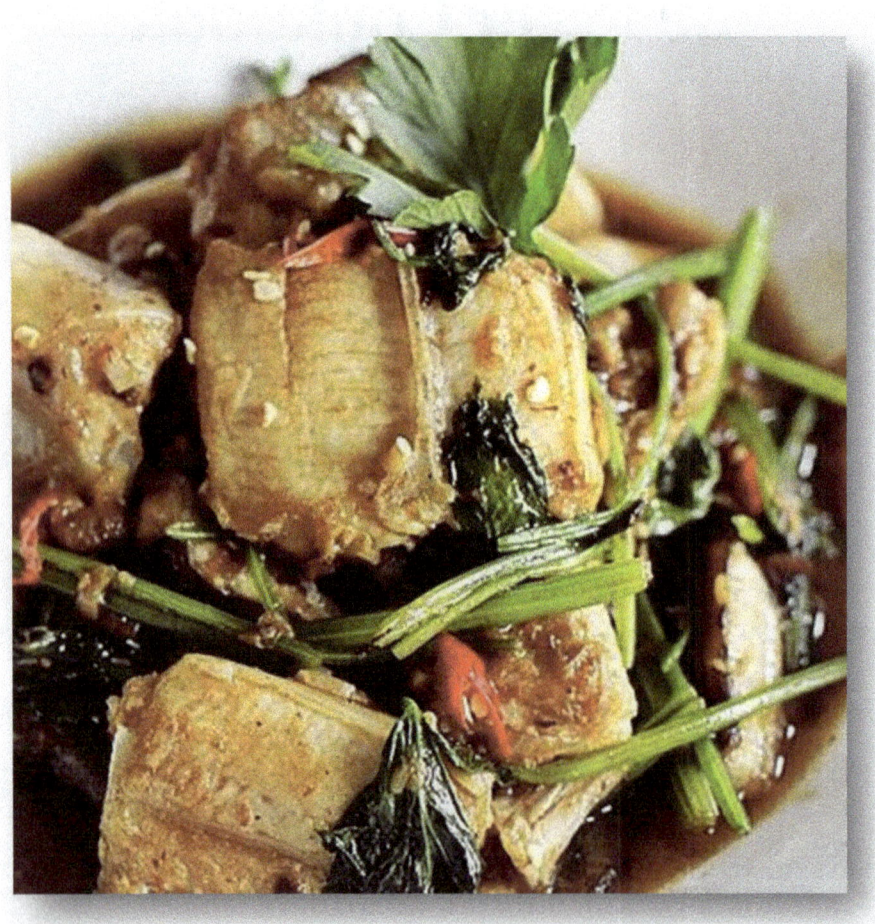

© copyright 2021 – all rights reserved.

the content contained within this book may not be reproduced, duplicated or transmitted without direct written permission from the author or the publisher.

under no circumstances will any blame or legal responsibility be held against the publisher, or author, for any damages, reparation, or monetary loss due to the information contained within this book. either directly or indirectly.

legal notice:

this book is copyright protected. this book is only for personal use. you cannot amend, distribute, sell, use, quote or paraphrase any part, or the content within this book, without the consent of the author or publisher.

disclaimer notice:

please note the information contained within this document is for educational and entertainment purposes only. all effort has been executed to present accurate, up to date, and reliable, complete information. no warranties of any kind are declared or implied. readers acknowledge that the author is not engaging in the rendering of legal, financial, medical or professional advice. the content within this book has been derived from various sources. please consult a licensed professional before attempting any techniques outlined in this book.

by reading this document, the reader agrees that under no circumstances is the author responsible for any losses, direct or indirect, which are incurred as a result of the use of information contained within this document, including, but not limited to, — errors, omissions, or inaccuracies.

Table of Contents

QUICK AND EASY RECIPES 6
- FRIED SQUASH FLOWERS 6
- SPINACH 8
- ZUCCHINI BLOOMS 9
- CHICKEN CHEESE FILLET 11
- PINEAPPLE PIZZA 13
- MACARONI CHEESE TOAST.. 15

BREAKFAST RECIPES...17
- AIR FRYER MEATBALLS IN TOMATO SAUCE........................... 17
- CHICKEN FRIED SPRING ROLLS 19
- MUSHROOM AND CHEESE FRITTATA.. 21
- CINNAMON AND CHEESE PANCAKE 23
- LOW-CARB WHITE EGG AND SPINACH FRITTATA............... 25
- SCALLION SANDWICH 27

SNACKS AND APPETIZER RECIPES 29
- SWEET POTATO FRIES 29
- CHEESE STICKS 32
- ZUCCHINI CRISPS 34
- TORTILLAS IN GREEN MANGO SALSA...................................... 36
- SKINNY PUMPKIN CHIPS 38
- PALM TREES HOLDER.. 40
- RIPE PLANTAINS 42

PORK, BEEF AND LAMB RECIPES... 44
- AIR FRYER STEAK.. 44
- PORK ON A BLANKET 46
- VIETNAMESE GRILLED PORK.. 48
- PROVENCAL RIBS 51
- AIR FRYER BEEF STEAK KABOBS WITH VEGETABLES...........53
- FRIED PORK CHOPS 55

PORK LIVER 57

FISH & SEAFOOD RECIPES **59**

SALMON CAKES IN AIR FRYER 59
COCONUT SHRIMP 61
CRISPY FISH STICKS IN AIR FRYER 64
HONEY-GLAZED SALMON 66

POULTRY RECIPES **68**

ROASTED VEGETABLE AND CHICKEN SALAD 68
CHICKEN SATAY 70
CHICKEN FAJITAS WITH AVOCADOS 72
CRISPY BUTTERMILK FRIED CHICKEN 74
GARLICKY CHICKEN WITH CREAMER POTATOES 76
BAKED CHICKEN CORDON BLEU 78

VEGETABLES AND SIDES RECIPES **80**

RAVIOLI 80
ONION RINGS 82
CAULIFLOWER FRITTERS 85
ZUCCHINI FRITTERS 87
KALE CHIPS 89
RADISH CHIPS 91
ZUCCHINI FRIES 93
AVOCADO FRIES 95

DESSERT RECIPES **97**

TASTY BANANA CAKE 97
SIMPLE CHEESECAKE 99
BREAD PUDDING 101
BREAD DOUGH AND AMARETTO DESSERT 103
WRAPPED PEARS 105
AIR FRIED BANANAS 107

QUICK AND EASY RECIPES

FRIED SQUASH FLOWERS

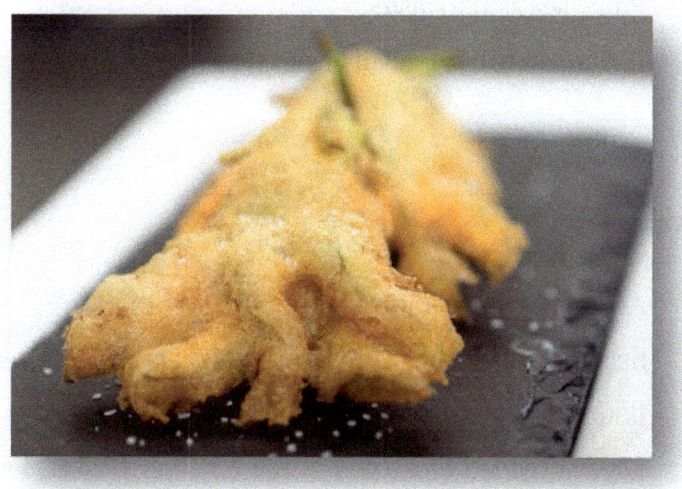

Preparation Time: 5 minutes

Cooking Time: 8 minutes

Servings: 3

Nutritional values:

- Calories: 5 kcal
- Carbohydrates: 1 g
- Fat: 0.1 g
- Proteins: 0.2 g

Ingredients:

- 2-½ lbs. rinsed squash flowers
- 1 cup coconut flour, finely milled
- Pinch sea salt, to taste
- Raisin vinegar for garnish, optional

Directions:

1. Adjust the temperature of the Air Fryer to 330°F.
2. Season squash blossoms with salt. Dredge into coconut flour.
3. Layer breaded blossoms in the air fryer basket. Fry for 2 minutes or until golden brown. Drain on paper towels.
4. Stack cooked squash blossoms in the middle of plates. Sprinkle raisin vinegar. Serve.

SPINACH

Preparation Time: 5 minutes

Cooking Time: 5 minutes

Servings: 3

Nutritional values:

- Calories: 81.6 kcal
- Carbohydrates: 4.5 g
- Fat: 6.9 g
- Proteins: 1.3 g

Ingredients:

- 2-½ lbs. fresh spinach leaves and tender stems only
- Sea salt

Directions:

1. Adjust the temperature of the Air Fryer to 330°F.
2. Put spinach in the Air fryer basket and fry for 20 seconds. Drain on paper towels. Repeat the step with the rest of the spinach. Season with salt. Serve.

ZUCCHINI BLOOMS

Preparation Time: 5 minutes

Cooking Time: 12 minutes

Servings: 3

Nutritional values:

- Calories: 117 kcal
- Carbohydrates: 8 g
- Fat: 8 g
- Proteins: 1 g

Ingredients:

- 2-½ lbs. rinsed zucchini flowers
- 1 cup fine-milled almond flour
- Sea salt
- Balsamic vinegar

Directions:

1. Adjust the temperature of the Air Fryer to 330°F.

2. Half-fill deep fryer with oil. Set this at medium heat. Lightly season zucchini flowers with salt, and then dredge in almond flour.
3. Layer breaded flowers into the Air Fryer basket.
4. Fry until golden brown. Drain on paper towels.
5. Transfer to a plate. Pour balsamic vinegar if using. Serve.

CHICKEN CHEESE FILLET

Preparation Time: 5 minutes

Cooking Time: 18 minutes

Servings: 4

Nutritional values:

- Calories: 386 kcal
- Fat: 21 g
- Carbohydrates: 14.3 g
- Proteins: 30 g

Ingredients:

- 2 chicken fillets
- 4 Gouda cheese slices
- 4 ham slices
- Salt and Pepper
- 1 tbsp. chopped chives

Directions:

1. Adjust the temperature of the air fryer to 180°C.
2. Cut chicken fillet into four pieces. Make a slit horizontally to the edge.
3. Open the fillet and season with salt and pepper.
4. Cover each piece with chives and cheese slices.
5. Close the fillet and wrap it in a ham slice.
6. Place wrap chicken fillet into an air fryer basket and cook for 15 minutes. Serve hot.

PINEAPPLE PIZZA

Preparation Time: 5 minutes

Cooking Time: 11 minutes

Servings: 3

Nutritional values:

- Calories: 80 kcal
- Fat: 2 g
- Carbohydrates: 12 g
- Proteins: 4 g

Ingredients:

- 1 whole wheat tortilla
- ¼ cup tomato pizza sauce
- ¼ cup pineapple tidbits
- ¼ cup grated mozzarella cheese
- ¼ cup ham slice

Directions:

1. Adjust the temperature of the air fryer to 300°F.

2. Place the tortilla on a baking sheet, then spread pizza sauce over the tortilla.
3. Arrange ham slice, cheese, and the pineapple over the tortilla.
4. Place the pizza in the air fryer basket and cook for 10 minutes. Serve hot.

MACARONI CHEESE TOAST

Preparation Time: 5 minutes

Cooking Time: 8 minutes

Servings: 2

Nutritional values:

- Calories: 250 kcal
- Fat: 16g
- Carbohydrates: 9 g
- Proteins: 14 g

Ingredients:

- 1 beaten egg
- 4 tbsp. Cheddar cheese
- Salt and pepper
- ½ cup macaroni and cheese
- 4 bread slices

Directions:

1. Spread the cheese, macaroni, and cheese over the two bread slices.

2. Place the other bread slices on top of the cheese and cut diagonally.
3. In a bowl, place the beaten egg and season with salt and pepper.
4. Brush the egg mixture onto the bread.
5. Place the bread into the air fryer and cook at 300°F for 5 minutes.

BREAKFAST RECIPES

AIR FRYER MEATBALLS IN TOMATO SAUCE

Preparation Time: 5 minutes

Cooking Time: 13 minutes

Servings: 4

Nutritional values:

- Calories: 129 kcal
- Fat: 17.8 g
- Carbohydrates: 15.4 g
- Proteins: 17.6 g

Ingredients:

- 1 egg
- 3/4 pound lean ground beef
- 1 onion, chopped
- 3 tbsp. breadcrumbs
- ½ tbsp. fresh thyme leaves, chopped

- ½ cup tomato sauce
- 1 tbsp. parsley, chopped
- Pinch salt
- Pinch pepper, to taste

Directions:

1. Preheat the Air Fryer to 390°F.
2. Place all ingredients in a bowl. Mix until well-combined. Divide mixture into 12 balls. Place in the cooking basket.
3. Cook meatballs for 8 minutes.
4. Put the cooked meatballs in an oven dish. Pour the tomato sauce on top. Put the oven dish inside the cooking basket of the Air Fryer.
5. Cook for 5 minutes at 330°F.

CHICKEN FRIED SPRING ROLLS

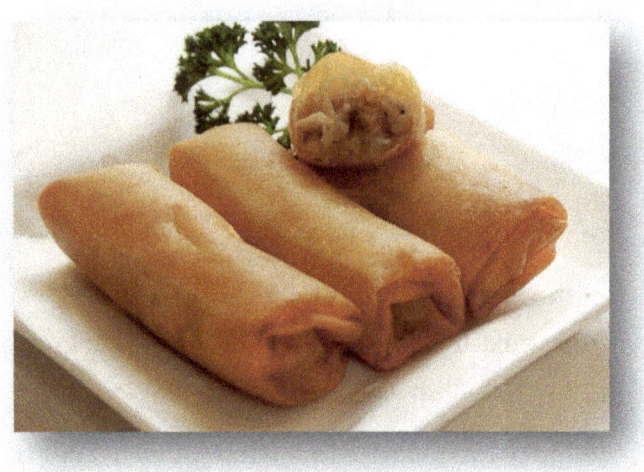

Preparation Time: 6 minutes

Cooking Time: 28 minutes

Servings: 4

Nutritional values:

- Calories: 150 kcal
- Fat: 5 g
- Carbohydrates: 18 g
- Proteins: 9 g

Ingredients:

For the spring roll wrappers:

- 1 egg, beaten
- 8 spring roll wrappers
- 1 tsp. cornstarch
- ½ tsp. olive oil

For the filling:

- 1 cup chicken breast, cooked, shredded
- 1 celery stalk, sliced thinly
- 1 carrot, sliced thinly
- 1 tsp. chicken stock powder, low sodium
- ½ tsp. ginger, chopped finely
- ½ cup sliced mushrooms

Directions:

1. Preheat the Air Fryer to 390°F.
2. Prepare the filling. In a bowl, combine shredded chicken, mushrooms, carrot, and celery. Add in chicken stock powder and ginger. Stir well.
3. Meanwhile, mix cornstarch and egg until thick in a bowl. Set aside.
4. Spoon some filling into a spring roll wrapper. Roll and seal the ends with the egg mixture.
5. Lightly brush spring rolls with oil and place them in the cooking basket. Cook for 20 minutes. Serve.

MUSHROOM AND CHEESE FRITTATA

Preparation Time: 7 minutes

Cooking Time: 20 minutes

Servings: 4

Nutritional values:

- Calories: 140 kcal
- Fat: 10.6 g
- Carbohydrates: 5.4 g
- Proteins: 22.7 g

Ingredients:

- 6 eggs
- 6 cups button mushrooms, sliced thinly
- 1 red onion, sliced into thin rounds
- 6 tbsp. feta cheese, reduced fat, crumbled
- Pinch salt
- 2 tbsp. olive oil

Directions:

1. Preheat Air Fryer to 330°F.
2. Sauté onions and mushrooms. Transfer to a plate with a paper towel.
3. Meanwhile, beat the eggs in a bowl. Season with salt. Coat a baking dish with cooking spray. Pour egg mixture.
4. Add in mushroom and onions. Top with crumbled feta cheese.
5. Place baking dish in the Air fryer basket. Cook for 20 minutes. Serve.

CINNAMON AND CHEESE PANCAKE

Preparation Time: 5 minutes

Cooking Time: 10 minutes

Servings: 4

Nutritional values:

- Calories: 140 kcal
- Fat: 10.6 g
- Carbohydrates: 5.4 g
- Proteins: 22.7 g

Ingredients:

- 2 eggs
- 2 cups cream cheese, reduced-fat
- ½ tsp. cinnamon
- 1 pack Stevia

Directions:

1. Preheat Air Fryer to 330°F.
2. Meanwhile, combine cream cheese, cinnamon, eggs, and stevia in a blender.
3. Pour ¼ of the mixture in the air fryer basket. Cook for 2 minutes on each side. Repeat the process with the rest of the mixture. Serve.

LOW-CARB WHITE EGG AND SPINACH FRITTATA

Preparation Time: 6 minutes

Cooking Time: 16 minutes

Servings: 4

Nutritional values:

- Calories: 120 kcal
- Fat: 4.5 g
- Carbohydrates: 13 g
- Proteins: 9.9 g

Ingredients:

- 8 egg whites
- 2 cups fresh spinach
- 2 tbsp. olive oil
- 1 green pepper, chopped
- 1 red pepper, chopped
- ½ cup feta cheese, reduced fat, crumbled

- ¼ yellow onion, chopped
- 1 tsp. salt
- 1 tsp. pepper

Directions:

1. Preheat the Air Fryer to 330°F.
2. Place red and green peppers and onions in the Air Fryer basket and cook for 3 minutes. Season with salt and pepper.
3. Pour egg whites and cook for 4 minutes. Add in the spinach and feta cheese on top.
4. Cook for 5 minutes.
5. Transfer to a plate. Slice and serve.

SCALLION SANDWICH

Preparation Time: 5 minutes

Cooking Time: 12 minutes

Servings: 1

Nutritional values:

- Calories: 154 kcal
- Fat: 2.5 g
- Carbohydrates: 9 g
- Proteins: 8.6 g

Ingredients:

- 2 slices wheat bread
- 2 tsp. butter, low fat
- 2 scallions, sliced thinly
- 1 tbsp. parmesan cheese, grated
- 3/4 cup cheddar cheese, reduced-fat, grated

Directions:

1. Preheat the Air fryer to 356°F.

2. Spread butter on a slice of bread. Place inside the cooking basket with the butter side facing down.
3. Place cheese and scallions on top. Spread the rest of the butter on the other slice of bread. Put it on top of the sandwich and sprinkle it with parmesan cheese.
4. Cook for 10 minutes.

SNACKS AND APPETIZER RECIPES

SWEET POTATO FRIES

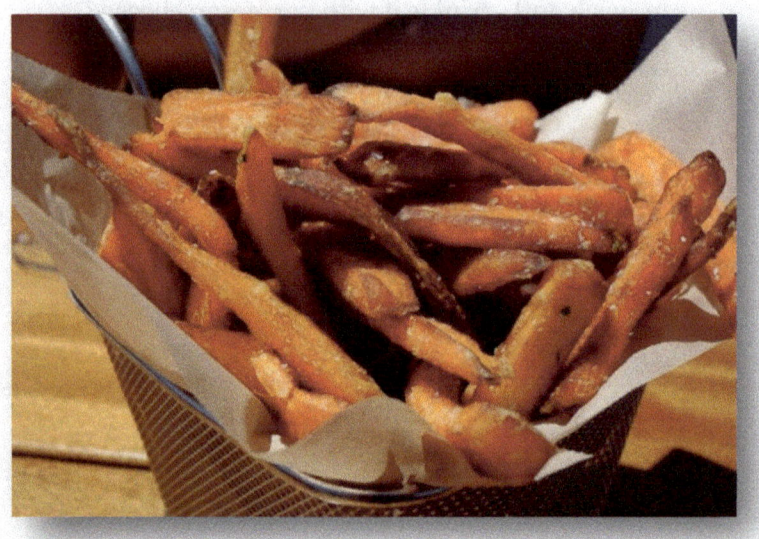

Preparation Time: 5 minutes

Cooking Time: 13 minutes

Servings: 4

Nutritional values:

- Calories: 130
- Fat: 2.3 g
- Carbohydrates: 27 g

- Proteins: 1.2 g

Ingredients:

- 2 medium sweet potatoes, peeled
- 1 tbsp. arrowroot starch
- 2 tbsp. cinnamon
- ¼ cup coconut sugar
- 2 tsp. melted butter, unsalted
- ½ tbsp. olive oil
- Confectioner's swerve as needed

Directions:

1. Switch on the Air Fryer, insert fryer basket, grease it with olive oil, then shut with its lid, set the fryer to 370°F, and preheat for 5 minutes.
2. Meanwhile, cut peeled sweet potatoes into ½-inch thick slices, place them in a bowl, add oil and starch and toss until well coated.
3. Open the fryer, add sweet potatoes to it, close with its lid, and cook for 8 minutes until nicely golden, shaking halfway through the frying.

4. When the Air Fryer beeps, open its lid, transfer sweet potato fries in a bowl, add butter, sprinkle with sugar and cinnamon and toss until well mixed.
5. Sprinkle confectioners swerve on the fries and serve.

CHEESE STICKS

Preparation Time: 5–7 minutes

Cooking Time: 10 minutes

Servings: 2

Nutritional values:

- Calories: 229
- Fat: 10 g
- Carbohydrates: 16 g
- Proteins: 15 g

Ingredients:

- 10 pieces spring roll wrappers, separated, quartered
- ¼ pound sharp cheddar cheese, reduced-fat, sliced into 2" x ½" matchsticks
- Oil for spraying

Directions:

1. Preheat the Air Fryer to 400°F.

2. Place cheese matchstick at the widest end of quartered spring roll wrapper. Moisten edges and tip of the wrapper with water. Fold spring roll wrapper over cheese, and tuck in both ends. Roll spring rolls tightly up to the tip. Place this into a freezer-safe container lined with saran wrap. Repeat the step for all cheese and spring roll wrappers.
3. Freeze for an hour before frying.
4. Spray a small amount of oil all over cheese matchsticks. Place a generous handful inside the Air Fryer basket. Fry for 3 to 5 minutes, or only until wrappers turn golden brown. Shake contents of the basket once midway through.
5. Remove from the basket. Set on plates. Repeat the step for the remaining breaded cheese sticks. Serve.

ZUCCHINI CRISPS

Preparation Time: 30 minutes

Cooking Time: 20 minutes

Servings: 2

Nutritional values:

- Calories: 15.2
- Fat: 0.1 g
- Carbohydrates: 3.6 g
- Proteins: 0.6 g

Ingredients:

- 2 zucchinis, sliced into a 1/8-inch-thick disk
- Pinch sea salt
- white pepper to taste
- olive oil for drizzling

Directions:

1. Preheat the Air Fryer to 330°F.

2. Put zucchini in a bowl with salt. Let it sit in a colander to drain for 30 minutes.
3. Layer zucchini in a baking dish. Drizzle in oil. Season with pepper. Place baking dish in the Air Fryer basket. Cook for 30 minutes.
4. Adjust seasoning. Serve.

TORTILLAS IN GREEN MANGO SALSA

Preparation Time: 30 minutes

Cooking Time: 10 minutes

Servings: 4

Nutritional values:

- Calories: 128 kcal
- Fat: 3.6 g
- Carbohydrates: 8.6 g
- Proteins: 2.7 g

Ingredients:

Tortillas:

- 4 pieces corn tortillas
- 1 tbsp. olive oil
- 1/16 tsp. sea salt

Green mango salsa:

- 1 green/unripe mango, minced
- 1 red/ripe Roma tomato, preferably minced
- 1 shallot, peeled, minced
- 1 fresh jalapeno pepper, minced
- ¼ red bell pepper, minced
- 4 tbsp. fresh cilantro, minced
- ¼ cup lime juice, freshly squeezed
- 1/16 tsp. salt

Directions:

1. Preheat the Air Fryer to 400°F.
2. Mix lime juice and salt in a bowl. Stir until solids dissolve. Add in the remaining salsa ingredients. Chill in the fridge for at least 30 minutes. Stir again just before using.
3. Lightly brush oil on both sides of tortillas. Cut these into large triangles.
4. Place a generous handful of sliced tortillas in the Air Fryer basket. Fry these for 10 minutes or until bread blisters and turns golden brown. Shake contents of the basket once midway through.
5. Place cooked pieces on a plate. Repeat step for remaining tortillas. Season with salt.
6. Place equal portions of crispy tortillas on plates. Serve with green mango and tomato salsa on the side.

SKINNY PUMPKIN CHIPS

Preparation Time: 20 minutes

Cooking Time: 10 minutes

Servings: 2

Nutritional values:

- Calories 118 kcal
- Fat: 14.7 g
- Carbohydrates: 2.2 g
- Proteins: 6.2 g

Ingredients:

- 1 pound pumpkin, cut into sticks
- 1 tbsp. coconut oil
- ½ tsp. rosemary
- ½ tsp. basil
- Salt and ground black pepper, to taste

Directions:

1. Start by preheating the Air Fryer to 395°F. Brush the pumpkin sticks with coconut oil; add the spices and toss to combine.
2. Cook for 13 minutes, shaking the basket halfway through the cooking time.
3. Serve with mayonnaise. Bon appétit!

PALM TREES HOLDER

Preparation Time: 5 minutes

Cooking Time: 15 minutes

Servings: 2

Nutritional values:

- Calories: 108 kcal
- Fat: 12 g
- Carbohydrates: 29 g
- Proteins: 4 g

Ingredients:

- 1 Sheet puff pastry
- Sugar

Directions:

1. Stretch the puff pastry sheet.
2. Pour the sugar over and fold the puff pastry sheet in half.

3. Put a thin layer of sugar on top and fold the puff pastry in half again.
4. Roll the puff pastry sheet from both ends towards the center (creating the palm tree's shape).
5. Cut into sheets 5–8 mm thick.
6. Preheat the Air Fryer to 180°C and put the palm trees in the basket.
7. Set the timer about 10 minutes at 180°C.

RIPE PLANTAINS

Preparation Time: 10 minutes

Cooking Time: 10 minutes

Servings: 2

Nutritional values:

- Calories: 209 kcal
- Fat: 8 g
- Carbohydrates: 29 g
- Proteins: 2.9 g

Ingredients:

- 2 pieces large ripe plantain, peeled, sliced into inch thick disks
- 1 tbsp. coconut butter, unsweetened

Directions:

1. Preheat the Air Fryer to 350°F.

2. Brush a small amount of coconut butter on all the sides of the plantain disks.
3. Place one even layer into the Air Fryer basket, making sure none overlap or touch. Fry plantains for 10 minutes.
4. Remove from the basket. Place on plates. Repeat the step for all the plantains.
5. While plantains are still warm. Serve.

PORK, BEEF AND LAMB RECIPES

AIR FRYER STEAK

Preparation Time: 6 minutes

Cooking Time: 15 minutes

Servings: 2

Nutritional values:

- Calories: 301 kcal
- Fat: 23 g
- Carbohydrates: 0 g
- Proteins: 23 g

Ingredients:

- 1 rib eye steak or New York City strip steak
- Salt and pepper
- Garlic powder
- Paprika
- Butter

Directions:

1. Place the meat to sit in a bowl at room temperature level.
2. Spray the olive oil onto both sides of the steak.
3. Add salt and pepper to season.
4. Add the garlic powder and paprika to the mixture.
5. Adjust the temperature of the air fryer to 400°F.
6. Place steak in the air fryer and cook for 12 minutes flipping it halfway through.
7. Lead it with butter when ready, then serve.

PORK ON A BLANKET

Preparation Time: 12 minutes

Cooking Time: 18 minutes

Servings: 4

Nutritional values:

- Calories: 242
- Fat: 14 g
- Carbohydrates: 0 g
- Proteins: 27 g

Ingredients:

- ½ puff defrosted pastry sheet
- 16 thick smoked sausages
- 15 ml milk

Directions:

1. Adjust the temperature of the air fryer to 200°C and set the timer to 5 minutes.

2. Cut the puff pastry into 64 x 38 mm strips.
3. Place a cocktail sausage at the end of the puff pastry and roll around the sausage, sealing the dough with some water.
4. Brush the top of the sausages wrapped in milk and place them in the preheated air fryer.
5. Cook at 200°C for 10 minutes or until golden brown.

VIETNAMESE GRILLED PORK

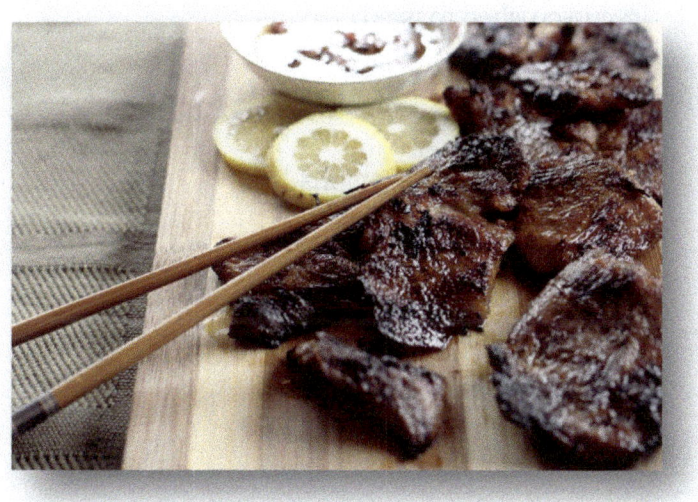

Preparation Time: 6 minutes

Cooking Time: 16 minutes

Servings: 6

Nutritional values:

- Calories: 231 kcal
- Fat: 16 g
- Carbohydrates: 4 g
- Proteins: 16 g

Ingredients:

- 1-pound sliced pork shoulder, pastured, fat trimmed
- 2 tbsp. chopped parsley
- ¼ cup crushed roasted peanuts

For the Marinade:

- ¼ cup minced white onions
- 1 tbsp. minced garlic
- 1 tbsp. lemongrass paste
- 1 tbsp. erythritol sweetener
- ½ tsp. ground black pepper
- 1 tbsp. fish sauce
- 2 tsp. soy sauce
- 2 tbsp. olive oil

Directions:

1. Place all the ingredients for the marinade in a bowl, stir well until combined and add it into a large plastic bag.
2. Cut the pork into ½-inch slices, cut each slice into 1-inches pieces, then add them into the plastic bag containing marinade, seal the bag, turn it upside down to coat the pork pieces with the marinade, and marinate for a minimum of 1 hour.

3. Then switch on the air fryer, insert fryer basket, grease it with olive oil, then shut with its lid, set the fryer at 400°F, and preheat for 5 minutes.
4. Open the fryer, add marinated pork in it in a single layer, close with its lid and cook for 10 minutes until nicely golden and cooked, flipping the pork halfway through the frying.
5. When the air fryer beeps, open its lid, transfer pork onto a serving plate, and keep warm.
6. Air fryer the remaining pork pieces in the same manner and then serve.

PROVENCAL RIBS

Preparation Time: 6 minutes

Cooking Time: 20-25 minutes

Servings: 4

Nutritional values:

- Calories: 296 kcal
- Fat: 22.63 g
- Carbohydrates: 0 g
- Proteins: 21.71 g

Ingredients:

- 500 g pork ribs
- Provencal herbs
- Salt
- Ground pepper
- Oil

Directions:

1. Put the ribs in a bowl and add some oil, Provencal herbs, salt, and ground pepper.
2. Stir well and leave in the fridge for at least 1 hour.
3. Put the ribs in the basket of the air fryer and select 200°C for 20 minutes.
4. From time to time, shake the basket and remove the ribs.

AIR FRYER BEEF STEAK KABOBS WITH VEGETABLES

Preparation Time: 9 minutes

Cooking Time: 11 minutes

Servings: 4

Nutritional values:

- Calories: 268 kcal
- Fat: 10 g
- Carbohydrates: 15 g
- Proteins: 20 g

Ingredients:

- Light soy sauce: 2 tbsp.
- Lean beef chuck ribs: 4 cups, cut into one-inch pieces
- Low-fat sour cream: 1/3 cup
- Half onion
- 8 skewers: 6 inches
- One bell pepper

Directions:

1. In a mixing bowl, add soy sauce and sour cream, mix well. Add the lean beef chunks, coat well, and let it marinate for half an hour or more.
2. Cut onion, bell pepper into one-inch pieces. In water, soak skewers for ten minutes.
3. Add onions, bell peppers, and beef on skewers; alternatively, sprinkle with black pepper.
4. Let it cook for 10 minutes in a preheated air fryer at 400°F, flip halfway through.
5. Serve with yogurt dipping sauce.

FRIED PORK CHOPS

Preparation Time: 9 minutes

Cooking Time: 38 minutes

Servings: 2

Nutritional values:

- Calories: 118 kcal
- Fat: 6.85 g
- Carbohydrates: 0 g
- Proteins: 13.12 g

Ingredients:

- 3 cloves ground garlic
- 2 tbsp. olive oil
- 1 tbsp. marinade
- 4 thawed pork chops

Directions:

1. In a bowl, mix the cloves of ground garlic, oil, and marinade.

2. Apply the mixture on the pork chops.
3. Put the chops in the air fryer and cook at 360°C for 35 minutes.

PORK LIVER

Preparation Time: 9 minutes

Cooking Time: 16 minutes

Servings: 4

Nutritional values:

- Calories: 120 kcal
- Fat: 3.41 g
- Carbohydrates: 0 g
- Proteins: 20.99 g

Ingredients:

- 500 g pork liver cut into steaks
- Breadcrumbs
- Salt
- Ground pepper
- 1 lemon
- Extra virgin olive oil

Directions:

1. Put the steaks on a plate or bowl.
2. Add the lemon juice, salt, and ground pepper.
3. Leave a few minutes to macerate the pork liver fillets.
4. Drain well and go through breadcrumbs; it is not necessary to pass the fillets through beaten egg because the liver is very moist, the breadcrumbs are perfectly glued.
5. Spray with extra virgin olive oil. If you don't have a sprayer, paint with a silicone brush.
6. Put the pork liver fillets in the air fryer basket.
7. Program 180°C, 10 minutes.
8. Take out if you see them golden to your liking and put another batch.
9. You should not pile the pork liver fillets, which are well extended so that the empanada is crispy on all sides.

FISH & SEAFOOD RECIPES

SALMON CAKES IN AIR FRYER

Preparation Time: 9 minutes

Cooking Time: 11 minutes

Servings: 2

Nutritional values:

- Calories: 194 kcal
- Fat: 9 g
- Carbohydrates: 1 g
- Proteins: 25 g

Ingredients:

- Fresh salmon fillet 8 oz.
- Egg 1
- Salt 1/8 tsp.
- Garlic powder ¼ tsp.
- Sliced lemon 1

Directions:

1. In the bowl, chop the salmon, add the egg and spices.
2. Form tiny cakes.
3. Let the Air fryer preheat to 390°F. On the bottom of the air fryer bowl lay sliced lemons—place cakes on top.
4. Cook them for seven minutes. Based on your diet preferences, eat with your chosen dip.

COCONUT SHRIMP

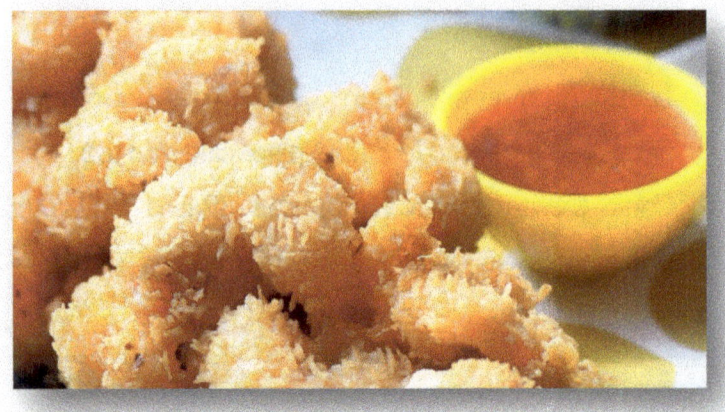

Preparation Time: 9 minutes

Cooking Time: 31 minutes

Servings: 4

Nutritional values:

- Calories: 340 kcal
- Proteins: 25 g
- Carbohydrates: 9 g
- Fat: 16g

Ingredients:

- Pork Rinds: ½ cup (Crushed)
- Jumbo shrimp: 4 cups. (deveined)
- Coconut flakes preferably: ½ cup
- Eggs: two
- Flour of coconut: ½ cup
- Any oil of your choice for frying at least half-inch in pan
- Freshly ground black pepper and kosher salt to taste

Dipping sauce:

- Powdered Sugar as Substitute: 2–3 tbsp.
- Mayonnaise: 3 tbsp.
- Sour Cream: ½ cup
- Coconut Extract or to taste: ¼ tsp.
- Coconut Cream: 3 tbsp.
- Pineapple Flavoring as much to taste: ¼ tsp.
- Coconut Flakes preferably unsweetened this is optional: 3 tbsp.

Directions:

Sauce

1. Mix all the ingredients into a tiny bowl for the Dipping sauce (Pina colada flavor). Combine well and put in the fridge until ready to serve.

Shrimps

2. Whip all eggs in a deep bowl and in a small shallow bowl; add the crushed pork rinds, coconut flour, sea salt, coconut flakes, and freshly ground black pepper.
3. Put the shrimp one by one in the mixed eggs for dipping, then in the coconut flour blend. Put them on a clean plate or put them on your air fryer's basket.
4. Place the shrimp battered in a single layer on your air fryer basket. Spritz the shrimp with oil and cook for 8–10 minutes at 360°F, flipping them through halfway.
5. Enjoy hot with dipping sauce.

CRISPY FISH STICKS IN AIR FRYER

Preparation Time: 9 minutes

Cooking Time: 16 minutes

Servings: 4

Nutritional values:

- Calories: 263 kcal
- Fat: 16g
- Carbohydrates: 1 g
- Proteins: 26.4 g

Ingredients:

- Whitefish such as cod 1 lb.
- Mayonnaise ¼ c
- Dijon mustard 2 tbsp.
- Water 2 tbsp.
- Pork rind 1&½ c
- Cajun seasoning ¾ tsp.

- Kosher salt and pepper to taste

Directions:

1. Spray non-stick cooking spray to the air fryer rack.
2. Pat the fish dry and cut into sticks about 1 inch by 2 inches' broad
3. Stir together the mayo, mustard, and water in a tiny small dish. Mix the pork rinds & Cajun seasoning into another small container.
4. Adding kosher salt and pepper to taste (both pork rinds and seasoning can have a decent amount of kosher salt, so you can dip a finger to see how salty it is).
5. Working for one slice of fish at a time, dip to cover in the mayo mix & then tap off the excess. Dip into the mixture of pork rind, then flip to cover. Place on the rack of an air fryer.
6. Set at 400F to Air Fry use for 5 minutes, then turn the fish with tongs and bake for another 5 minutes. Serve.

HONEY-GLAZED SALMON

Preparation Time: 11 minutes

Cooking Time: 16 minutes

Servings: 2

Nutritional values:

- Calories: 254 kcal
- Fat: 12 g
- Carbohydrates: 9.9 g
- Proteins: 20 g

Ingredients:

- Gluten-free soy sauce: 6 tsp.
- Salmon fillets: 2 pcs
- Sweet rice wine: 3 tsp.
- Water: 1 tsp.
- Honey: 6 tbsp.

Directions:

1. In a bowl, mix sweet rice wine, soy sauce, honey, and water.
2. Set half of it aside.
3. In half of it, marinate the fish and let it rest for two hours.
4. Let the air fryer preheat to 180°C
5. Cook the fish for 8 minutes, flip halfway through and cook for another five minutes.
6. Baste the salmon with marinade mixture after 3 or 4 minutes.
7. The half of marinade, pour in a saucepan, reduce to half, serve with a sauce.

POULTRY RECIPES

ROASTED VEGETABLE AND CHICKEN SALAD

Preparation Time: 9 minutes

Cooking Time: 13 minutes

Servings: 4

Nutritional values:

- Calories: 495 kcal
- Fat: 23 g
- Carbohydrates: 18 g
- Proteins: 51 g

Ingredients:

- 3 boneless, skinless chicken breasts, cut into 1-inch cubes
- 1 small red onion, sliced
- 1 orange bell pepper, sliced
- 1 cup sliced yellow summer squash
- 4 tbsp. honey mustard salad dressing, divided

- ½ tsp. dried thyme
- ½ cup mayonnaise
- 2 tbsp. freshly squeezed lemon juice

Directions:

1. Place the chicken, onion, pepper, and squash in the air fryer basket. Drizzle with 1 tbsp. of the honey mustard salad dressing, add the thyme and toss.
2. Roast at 400°F (204°C) for 10 to 13 minutes or until the chicken is 165°F (74°C) on a food thermometer, tossing the food once during cooking time.
3. Transfer the chicken and vegetables to a bowl and mix in the remaining 3 tbsp. of honey mustard salad dressing, the mayonnaise, and lemon juice. Serve on lettuce leaves, if desired.

CHICKEN SATAY

Preparation Time: 12 minutes

Cooking Time: 10-15 minutes

Servings: 4

Nutritional values:

- Calories: 449 kcal
- Carbohydrates: 8 g
- Fat: 28 g
- Proteins: 46 g

Ingredients:

- ½ cup crunchy peanut butter
- 1/3 cup chicken broth
- 3 tbsp. low-sodium soy sauce
- 2 tbsp. freshly squeezed lemon juice
- 2 cloves garlic, minced
- 2 tbsp. olive oil
- 1 tsp. curry powder
- 1 pound (454 g) chicken tenders

Directions:

1. In a medium bowl, combine the peanut butter, chicken broth, soy sauce, lemon juice, garlic, olive oil, and curry powder, and mix well with a wire whisk until smooth. Remove 2 tbsp. of this mixture into a small bowl. Put the remaining sauce into a serving bowl and set aside.
2. Add the chicken tenders to the bowl with the 2 tablespoons sauce and stir to coat. Let stand for a few minutes to marinate, then run a bamboo skewer through each chicken tender lengthwise.
3. Put the chicken in the air fryer basket and air fry in batches at 390°F (199°C) for 6 to 9 minutes or until the chicken reaches 165°F (74°C) on a meat thermometer. Serve the chicken with the reserved sauce.

CHICKEN FAJITAS WITH AVOCADOS

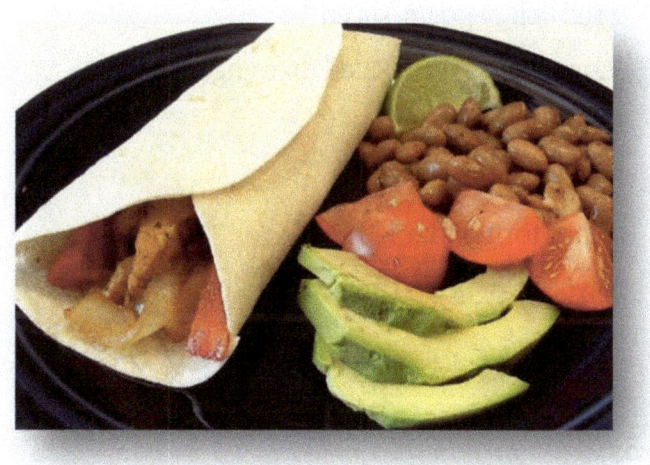

Preparation Time: 9 minutes

Cooking Time: 14 minutes

Servings: 4

Nutritional values:

- Calories: 784 kcal
- Fat: 38 g
- Carbohydrates: 39 g
- Proteins: 72 g

Ingredients:

- 4 boneless, skinless chicken breasts, sliced
- 1 small red onion, sliced
- 2 red bell peppers, sliced
- ½ cup spicy ranch salad dressing, divided
- ½ tsp. dried oregano
- 8 corn tortillas
- 2 cups torn butter lettuce
- 2 avocados, peeled and chopped

Directions:

1. Place the chicken, onion, and pepper in the air fryer basket. Drizzle with 1 tbsp. of the salad dressing and add the oregano. Toss to combine.
2. Air fry at 380°F (193°C) for 10 to 14 minutes or until the chicken is 165°F (74°C) on a food thermometer.
3. Transfer the chicken and vegetables to a bowl and toss with the remaining salad dressing.
4. Serve the chicken mixture with the tortillas, lettuce, and avocados and let everyone make their own creations.

CRISPY BUTTERMILK FRIED CHICKEN

Preparation Time: 8 minutes

Cooking Time: 28 minutes

Servings: 4

Nutritional values:

- Calories: 645 kcal
- Fat: 17 g
- Carbohydrates: 55 g
- Proteins: 62 g

Ingredients:

- 6 chicken pieces: drumsticks, breasts, and thighs
- 1 cup flour
- 2 tsp. paprika
- Pinch salt
- Freshly ground black pepper, to taste
- 1/3 cup buttermilk

- 2 eggs
- 2 tbsp. olive oil
- 1½ cups bread crumbs

Directions:

1. Pat the chicken dry. In a shallow bowl, combine the flour, paprika, salt, and pepper.
2. In another bowl, beat the buttermilk with the eggs until smooth.
3. In a third bowl, combine the olive oil and bread crumbs until mixed.
4. Dredge the chicken in the flour, then into the eggs to coat, and finally into the bread crumbs, patting the crumbs firmly onto the chicken skin.
5. Air fry the chicken at 370°F (188°C) for 20 to 25 minutes, turning each piece over halfway during cooking until the meat registers 165°F (74°C) on a meat thermometer and the chicken is brown and crisp. Let cool for 5 minutes, then serve.

GARLICKY CHICKEN WITH CREAMER POTATOES

Preparation Time: 11 minutes

Cooking Time: 20-25 minutes

Servings: 4

Nutritional values:

- Calories: 492 kcal
- Fat: 14 g
- Carbohydrates: 20 g
- Proteins: 68 g

Ingredients:

- 1 (2½- to 3-pound / 1.1- to 1.4-kg) broiler-fryer whole chicken
- 2 tbsp. olive oil
- ½ tsp. garlic salt
- 8 cloves garlic, peeled
- 1 slice lemon

- ½ tsp. dried thyme
- ½ tsp. dried marjoram
- 12 to 16 creamer potatoes, scrubbed

Directions:

1. Do not wash the chicken before cooking. Remove it from its packaging and pat the chicken dry.
2. Combine the olive oil and salt in a small bowl. Rub half of this mixture on the inside of the chicken, under the skin, and on the chicken skin. Place the garlic cloves and lemon slices inside the chicken. Sprinkle the chicken with thyme and marjoram.
3. Put the chicken in the air fryer basket. Surround with the potatoes and drizzle the potatoes with the remaining olive oil mixture.
4. Roast at 380°F (193°C) for 25 minutes, then test the temperature of the chicken. It should be 160°F (71°C). Test at the thickest part of the breast, making sure the probe doesn't touch bone. If the chicken isn't done yet, return it to the air fryer, roast it for 4 to 5 minutes, or until the temperature is 160°F (71°C).
5. When the chicken is done, transfer it and the potatoes to a serving platter and cover with foil. Let the chicken rest for 5 minutes before serving.

BAKED CHICKEN CORDON BLEU

Preparation Time: 15 minutes

Cooking Time: 13 minutes

Servings: 4

Nutritional values:

- Calories: 479 kcal
- Fat: 12 g
- Carbohydrates: 26 g
- Proteins: 64 g

Ingredients:

- 4 chicken breast fillets
- ¼ cup chopped ham
- 1/3 cup grated Swiss or Gruyere cheese
- ¼ cup flour
- Pinch salt
- Freshly ground black pepper, to taste

- ½ tsp. dried marjoram
- 1 egg
- 1 cup whole-wheat bread crumbs
- Olive oil for misting

Directions:

1. Put the chicken breast fillets on a work surface and gently press them with the palm of your hand to make them a bit thinner. Don't tear the meat.
2. In a small bowl, combine the ham and cheese. Divide this mixture among the chicken fillets. Wrap the chicken around the filling to enclose it, using toothpicks to hold the chicken together.
3. In a shallow bowl, mix the flour, salt, pepper, and marjoram. In another bowl, beat the egg. Spread the bread crumbs out on a plate.
4. Dip the chicken into the flour mixture, then into the egg, then into the bread crumbs to coat thoroughly.
5. Put the chicken in the air fryer basket and mist with olive oil.
6. Bake at 380°F (193°C) for 13 to 15 minutes or until the chicken is thoroughly cooked to 165°F (74°C). Carefully remove the toothpicks and serve.

VEGETABLES AND SIDES RECIPES

RAVIOLI

Preparation Time: 5 minutes

Cooking Time: 16 minutes

Servings: 4

Nutritional values:

- Calories: 150 kcal
- Fat: 3 g
- Carbohydrates: 27 g

Ingredients:

- 8 ounces frozen vegan ravioli, thawed
- 1 tsp. dried basil
- 1 tsp. garlic powder
- 1/8 tsp. ground black pepper
- ¼ tsp. salt
- 1 tsp. dried oregano
- 2 tsp. Nutritional yeast flakes

- ½ cup marinara sauce, unsweetened
- ½ cup panko bread crumbs
- ¼ cup liquid from chickpeas can

Directions:

1. Place breadcrumbs in a bowl, sprinkle with salt, basil, oregano, and black pepper, add garlic powder and yeast and stir until mixed.
2. Take a bowl and then pour in chickpeas liquid in it.
3. Working on one ravioli at a time, first dip a ravioli in chickpeas liquid and then coat with breadcrumbs mixture.
4. Prepare remaining ravioli in the same manner, then take a fryer basket, grease it well with oil, and place ravioli in it in a single layer.
5. Switch on the air fryer, insert fryer basket, sprinkle oil on ravioli, shut with its lid, set the fryer at 390°F, then cook for 6 minutes, turn the ravioli, and continue cooking 2 minutes until nicely golden and heated thoroughly.
6. Cook the remaining ravioli in the same manner and serve with marinara sauce.

ONION RINGS

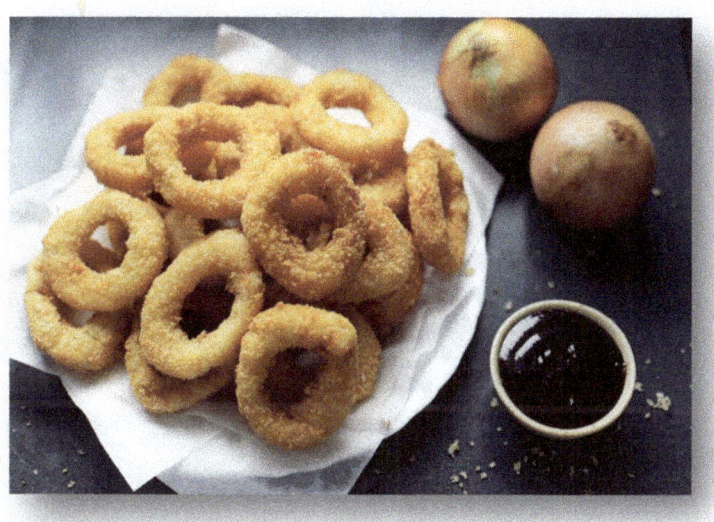

Preparation Time: 10 minutes

Cooking Time: 20 minutes

Servings: 4

Nutritional values:

- Calories: 135 kcal
- Fat: 7 g
- Carbohydrates: 8 g
- Proteins: 8 g

Ingredients:

- 1 large white onion, peeled
- 2/3 cup pork rinds
- 3 tbsp. almond flour
- ½ tsp. garlic powder
- ½ tsp. paprika
- ¼ tsp. sea salt
- 3 tbsp. coconut flour
- 2 eggs, pastured

Directions:

1. Switch on the air fryer, insert fryer basket, grease it with olive oil, then shut with its lid, set the fryer at 400°F and preheat for 10 minutes.
2. Meanwhile, slice the peeled onion into ½ inch thick rings.
3. Take a shallow dish, add almond flour, and stir in garlic powder, paprika, and pork rinds; take another shallow dish, add coconut flour, and salt and stir until mixed.
4. Crack eggs in a bowl and then whisk until combined.
5. Working on one onion ring at a time, first coat onion ring in coconut flour mixture, then it in egg, and coat with pork rind mixture by scooping over the onion until evenly coated.
6. Open the fryer, place coated onion rings in it in a single layer, spray oil over onion rings, close with its lid and cook

for 16 minutes until nicely golden and thoroughly cooked, flipping the onion rings halfway through the frying.
7. When the air fryer beeps, open its lid, transfer onion rings onto a serving plate and cook the remaining onion rings in the same manner.
8. Serve straight away.

CAULIFLOWER FRITTERS

Preparation Time: 10 minutes

Cooking Time: 14 minutes

Servings: 2

- **Nutritional values:**
- Calories: 272 kcal
- Fat: 0.3 g
- Carbohydrates: 57 g
- Proteins: 11 g

Ingredients:

- 5 cups chopped cauliflower florets
- ½ cup almond flour
- ½ tsp. baking powder
- ½ tsp. ground black pepper
- ½ tsp. salt
- 2 eggs, pastured

Directions:

1. Add chopped cauliflower in a blender or food processor, pulse until minced, and then tip the mixture in a bowl.
2. Add remaining ingredients, stir well and then shape the mixture into 1/3-inch patties, an ice cream scoop of mixture per patty.
3. Switch on the air fryer, insert fryer basket, grease it with olive oil, then shut with its lid, set the fryer at 390°F and preheat for 5 minutes.
4. Then open the fryer, add cauliflower patties in it in a single layer, spray oil over patties, close with its lid and cook for 14 minutes at 375°F until nicely golden and cooked, flipping the patties halfway through the frying.
5. Serve straight away with the dip.

ZUCCHINI FRITTERS

Preparation Time: 20 minutes

Cooking Time: 12 minutes

Servings: 4

Nutritional values:

- Calories: 57 kcal
- Fat: 1 g
- Carbohydrates: 8 g
- Proteins: 3 g

Ingredients:

- 2 medium zucchinis, ends trimmed
- 3 tbsp. almond flour
- 1 tbsp. salt
- 1 tsp. garlic powder
- ¼ tsp. paprika
- ¼ tsp. ground black pepper
- ¼ tsp. onion powder
- 1 egg, pastured

Directions:

1. Wash and pat dry the zucchini, then cut its ends and grate the zucchini.
2. Place grated zucchini in a colander, sprinkle with salt and let it rest for 10 minutes.
3. Then, wrap zucchini in a kitchen cloth, squeeze moisture from it as much as possible, and place dried zucchini in another bowl.
4. Add remaining ingredients into the zucchini and then stir until mixed.
5. Take the fryer basket, line it with parchment paper, grease it with oil, drop zucchini mixture on it by a spoonful, about 1-inch apart, and then spray well with oil.
6. Switch on the air fryer, insert fryer basket, then shut with its lid, set the fryer at 360°F and cook the fritter for 12 minutes until nicely golden and cooked, flipping the fritters halfway through the frying.
7. Serve straight away.

KALE CHIPS

Preparation Time: 5 minutes

Cooking Time: 7 minutes

Servings: 2

Nutritional values:

- Calories: 66.2 kcal
- Fat: 4 g
- Carbohydrates: 7.3 g
- Proteins: 2.5 g

Ingredients:

- 1 large bunch kale
- ¾ tsp. red chili powder
- 1 tsp. salt
- ¾ tsp. ground black pepper

Directions:

1. Remove the hard spines from the kale leaves, then cut kale into small pieces and place them in a fryer basket.
2. Spray oil over kale, then sprinkle with salt, chili powder, and black pepper and toss until well mixed.
3. Switch on the air fryer, insert fryer basket, then shut with its lid, set the fryer at 375°F and cook for 7 minutes until kale is crispy, shaking halfway through the frying.
4. When the air fryer beeps, open its lid, transfer kale chips onto a serving plate and serve.

RADISH CHIPS

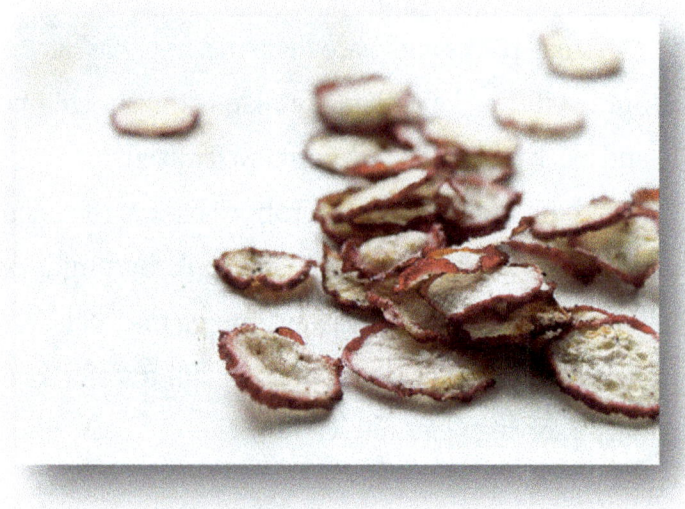

Preparation Time: 5 minutes

Cooking Time: 20 minutes

Servings: 2

Nutritional values:

- Calories: 21 kcal
- Fat: 1.8 g
- Carbohydrates: 1 g
- Proteins: 0.2 g

Ingredients:

- 8 ounces radish slices
- ½ tsp. garlic powder
- 1 tsp. salt
- ½ tsp. onion powder
- ½ tsp. ground black pepper

Directions:

1. Wash the radish slices, pat them dry, place them in a fryer basket, and then spray oil on them until well coated.
2. Sprinkle salt, garlic powder, onion powder, and black pepper over radish slices and then toss until well coated.
3. Switch on the air fryer, insert fryer basket, then shut with its lid, set the fryer at 370°F and cook for 10 minutes, stirring the slices halfway through.
4. Then spray oil on radish slices, shake the basket and continue frying for 10 minutes, stirring the chips halfway through.
5. Serve straight away.

ZUCCHINI FRIES

Preparation Time: 10 minutes

Cooking Time: 20 minutes

Servings: 4

Nutritional values:

- Calories: 147 kcal
- Fat: 10 g
- Carbohydrates: 6 g
- Proteins: 9 g

Ingredients:

- 2 medium zucchinis
- ½ cup almond flour
- 1/8 tsp. ground black pepper
- ½ tsp. garlic powder
- 1/8 tsp. salt
- 1 tsp. Italian seasoning
- ½ cup grated parmesan cheese, reduced-fat
- 1 egg, pastured, beaten

Directions:

1. Switch on the air fryer, insert fryer basket, grease it with olive oil, then shut with its lid, set the fryer at 400°F and preheat for 10 minutes.
2. Meanwhile, cut each zucchini in half and then cut each zucchini half into 4-inch-long pieces, each about ½-inch thick.
3. Place flour in a shallow dish, add remaining ingredients except for the egg and stir until mixed.
4. Crack the egg in a bowl and then whisk until blended.
5. Working on one zucchini piece at a time, first dip it in the egg, then coat it in the almond flour mixture and place it on a wire rack.
6. Open the fryer, add zucchini pieces in it in a single layer, spray oil over zucchini, close with its lid and cook for 10 minutes until nicely golden and crispy, shaking halfway through the frying.
7. Cook remaining zucchini pieces in the same manner and serve.

AVOCADO FRIES

Preparation Time: 10 minutes

Cooking Time: 20 minutes

Servings: 2

Nutritional values:

- Calories: 251 kcal
- Fat: 17 g
- Carbohydrates: 19 g
- Proteins: 6 g

Ingredients:

- 1 medium avocado, pitted
- 1 egg
- ½ cup almond flour
- ¼ tsp. salt
- ¼ tsp. ground black pepper
- ½ tsp. salt

Directions:

1. Switch on the air fryer, insert fryer basket, grease it with olive oil, then shut with its lid, set the fryer at 400°F and preheat for 10 minutes.
2. Meanwhile, cut the avocado in half and then cut each half into wedges, each about ½-inch thick.
3. Place flour in a shallow dish, add salt and black pepper, and stir until mixed.
4. Crack the egg in a bowl and then whisk until blended.
5. Working on one avocado piece at a time, first dip it in the egg, then coat it in the almond flour mixture and place it on a wire rack.
6. Open the fryer, add avocado pieces in a single layer, spray oil over avocado, close with its lid and cook for 10 minutes until nicely golden and crispy, shaking halfway through the frying.
7. When the air fryer beeps, open its lid, transfer avocado fries onto a serving plate and serve.

DESSERT RECIPES

TASTY BANANA CAKE

Preparation Time: 40 minutes

Cooking Time: 30 minutes

Servings: 4

Nutritional values:

- Calories: 145 kcal
- Fat: 16 g
- Carbohydrates: 9 g
- Proteins: 4 g

Ingredients:

- 1 tbsp. butter, soft
- 1 egg
- 1/3 cup brown sugar
- 2 tbsp. honey
- 1 banana
- 1 cup white flour

- 1 tbsp. baking powder
- ½ tbsp. cinnamon powder
- Cooking spray

Directions:

1. Spurt cake pan with cooking spray.
2. Mix in butter with honey, sugar, banana, cinnamon, egg, flour, and baking powder in a bowl, then beat.
3. Empty mix in a cake pan with cooking spray, put into the air fryer, and cook at 350°F for 30 minutes.
4. Allow for cooling, slice.
5. Serve.

SIMPLE CHEESECAKE

Preparation Time: 25 minutes

Cooking Time: 20 minutes

Servings: 15

Nutritional values:

- Calories: 149 kcal
- Fat: 11 g
- Carbohydrates: 3 g
- Proteins: 9 g

Ingredients:

- 1 lb. cream cheese
- ½ tbsp. vanilla extract
- 2 eggs
- 4 tbsp. sugar
- 1 cup graham crackers
- 2 tbsp. butter

Directions:

1. Mix in butter with crackers in a bowl.

2. Compress crackers blend to the bottom cake pan, put into the air fryer and cook at 350°F for 4 minutes.
3. Mix cream cheese with sugar, vanilla, egg in a bowl and beat properly.
4. Sprinkle filling on crackers crust and cook the cheesecake in the air fryer at 310°F for 15 minutes.
5. Keep cake in the fridge for 3 hours, slice.
6. Serve.

BREAD PUDDING

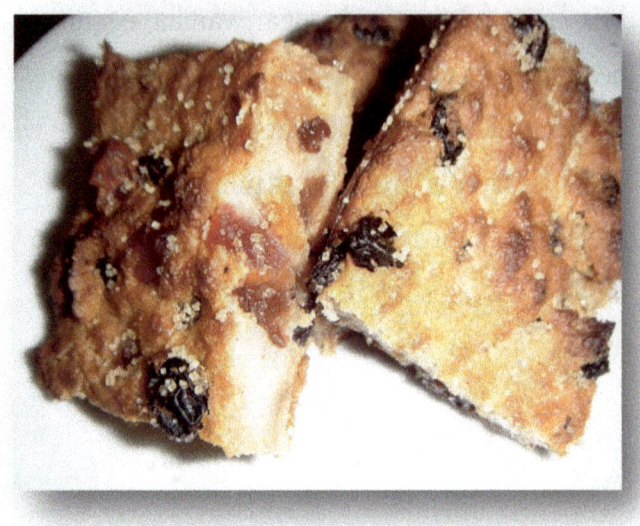

Preparation Time: 10 minutes

Cooking Time: 60 minutes

Servings: 4

Nutritional values:

- Calories: 139 kcal
- Fat: 11 g
- Carbohydrates: 7 g
- Proteins: 14 g

Ingredients:

- 6 glazed donuts
- 1 cup cherries
- 4 egg yolks
- 1 and ½ cups whipping cream
- ½ cup raisins
- ¼ cup sugar
- ½ cup chocolate chips

Directions:

1. Mix in cherries with whipping cream and egg in a bowl, then turn properly.
2. Mix in raisins with chocolate chips, sugar, and doughnuts in a bowl, then stir.
3. Mix the 2 mixtures, pour into an oiled pan, then into air fryer and cook at 310°F for 1 hour.
4. Cool pudding before cutting.
5. Serve.

BREAD DOUGH AND AMARETTO DESSERT

Preparation Time: 22 minutes

Cooking Time: 10-15 minutes

Servings: 12

Nutritional values:

- Calories: 165 kcal
- Fat: 11 g
- Carbohydrates: 9 g
- Proteins: 27 g

Ingredients:

- 1 lb. bread dough
- 1 cup sugar
- ½ cup butter
- 1 cup heavy cream
- 12 oz. chocolate chips
- 2 tbsp. amaretto liqueur

Directions:

1. Turn dough, cut into 20 slices, and cut each piece in halves.
2. Sweep dough pieces with spray sugar, butter, put into the air fryer's basket, and cook them at 350°F for 5 minutes. Turn them, cook for 3 minutes still. Move to a platter.
3. Melt the heavy cream in a pan over medium heat, put chocolate chips and turn until they melt.
4. Put in liqueur, turn, and move to a bowl.
5. Serve bread dippers with the sauce.

WRAPPED PEARS

Preparation Time: 10 minutes

Cooking Time: 16 minutes

Servings: 4

- **Nutritional values:**
- Calories: 169 kcal
- Fat: 19 g
- Carbohydrates: 5 g
- Proteins: 4 g

Ingredients:

- 4 puff pastry sheets
- 14 oz. vanilla custard
- 2 pears
- 1 egg
- ½ tbsp. cinnamon powder
- 2 tbsp. sugar

Directions:

1. Put wisp pastry slices on a flat surface, add a spoonful of vanilla custard at the center of each, add pear halves and wrap.
2. Sweep pears with egg, cinnamon, and spray sugar, put into the air fryer's basket, and cook at 320°F for 15 minutes.
3. Split parcels on plates.
4. Serve.

AIR FRIED BANANAS

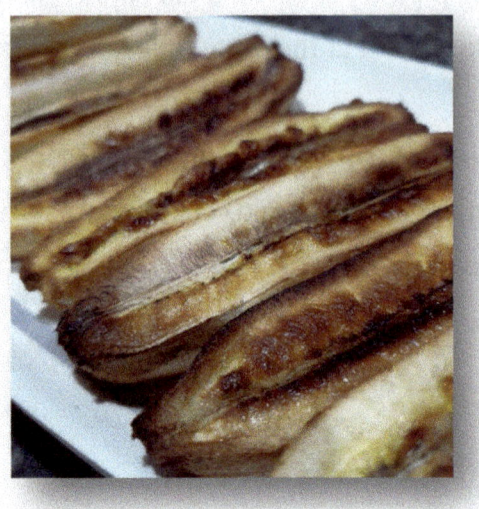

Preparation Time: 10 minutes

Cooking Time: 14 minutes

Servings: 4

Nutritional values:

- Calories: 166 kcal
- Fat: 11 g
- Carbohydrates: 9 g
- Proteins: 4 g

Ingredients:

- 3 tbsp. butter
- 2 eggs
- 8 bananas
- ½ cup corn flour
- 3 tbsp. cinnamon sugar
- 1 cup panko

Directions:

1. Warm-up the pan with the butter over medium heat, put panko, turn, and cook for 4 minutes then move to a bowl.
2. Spin each in flour, panko, egg blend, assemble them in the air fryer's basket, grime with cinnamon sugar and cook at 280°F for 10 minutes.
3. Serve immediately.

www.ingramcontent.com/pod-product-compliance
Lightning Source LLC
Chambersburg PA
CBHW070725030426
42336CB00013B/1924